Rafaela Reyes Garcia
Mabel Adela Perez Gonzalez
Ignasio Espinosa Perez

Adolescent Pregnancy Control Education Program

Rafaela Reyes Garcia
Mabel Adela Perez Gonzalez
Ignasio Espinosa Perez

Adolescent Pregnancy Control Education Program

Social, economic, school and psychological problem

ScienciaScripts

Imprint

Cover image: www.ingimage.com

This book is a translation from the original published under ISBN 978-620-2-14921-1.

Publisher:
Sciencia Scripts
is a trademark of
Dodo Books Indian Ocean Ltd. and OmniScriptum S.R.L publishing group

120 High Road, East Finchley, London, N2 9ED, United Kingdom
Str. Armeneasca 28/1, office 1, Chisinau MD-2012, Republic of Moldova, Europe
Printed at: see last page
ISBN: 978-620-7-88121-5

Contents

Summary

Introduction: Early adolescent pregnancy is a worldwide concern, especially for developing nations. **Objective**: To determine the effectiveness of an educational programme in adolescents for the control of modifiable risk factors associated with adolescent pregnancy at the Esperanza Medical Clinic #5 in the period February 2020-February 2022. **Methods:** A quasi-experimental longitudinal intervention study was carried out without a control group, prospectively in the Family Medical Clinic #5 of the Mario Muñoz Monroy polyclinic in the town of Esperanza. 35 female adolescents. Population 35 patients and sample 24. **Results:** There is a significant predominance of patients in the late adolescent stage, 54.2%, 79.2% of the adolescents with pre-university level, 79.2%, first sexual relations, 15 year olds (45.8%) and cohabiting partners (29.2%), no abortions (58%), economic difficulties (17%), no family history (54.1%), no sexually transmitted infections (75%), the factors that were modified were: alcohol consumption, family function, family function, use of alcohol, alcoholism, alcoholism, alcoholism, alcoholism, alcoholism, alcoholism, alcoholism, alcoholism, alcoholism, family function, alcoholism, alcoholism, alcoholism, alcoholism, family function, family function, alcoholism, family function, family function, family function, family function, family function, family function: alcohol consumption, family function, contraceptive use and very significant changes in the level of information in a positive way **Conclusions**: The proposed educational programme is effective.

Keywords: adolescent pregnancy, risk factors, educational programme

1 INTRODUCTION

Early adolescent pregnancy is a global concern, especially for developing nations. The consequences of pregnancy affect adolescents and their families, who often experience it as a conflict. For adolescent parents, the consequences are manifested at social, economic, educational and psychological levels, such as increased stress and greater frequency of emotional disturbances, working instead of studying, progressive abandonment of friends and time for leisure, as well as assuming a new role and having to act as an adult. (1, 2)

Adolescent pregnancy is considered a non-normative developmental crisis of a mixed nature as it increases stressful situations and disorganises the subject's life, however, for adolescents it can also mean a reason to live, to change their behaviour, to become more responsible, becoming a motivation to fight and to move forward. Adolescent pregnancy remains one of the main factors contributing to maternal and infant mortality, and to the cycle of disease and poverty (3).

The main objectives of comprehensive care for adolescents should be to achieve their maximum overall development, to contribute to their proper education and to detect any hidden disorders or illnesses early. Knowledge and management of risk factors (including early detection of circumstances such as pregnancy) are important (2).

The importance of social, cultural and economic conditions associated with adolescent pregnancy has been noted, including early marriage, low parental and adolescent schooling, deprivation and sexual abuse, all of which contribute to perpetuating the cycle of poverty. Moreover, lack of access to health services and contraceptive methods is a major barrier to preventing adolescent pregnancy. (1)

In Mexico, the National Strategy for the Prevention of Adolescent Pregnancy (ENAPEA) was implemented with five levels of intervention: influencing social determinants, improving the context to achieve healthy decisions, comprehensive sexual education, effective access to contraceptive methods and efficient clinical interventions. (4)

On the other hand, the Mexican Social Security Institute (IMSS) has developed sexual and reproductive health education strategies through the JUVENIMSS programme. However, the adolescent fertility rate (AFR) has not decreased significantly in recent years and Mexico ranks first in adolescent pregnancy among the member countries of the Organisation for Economic Co-operation and Development (OECD). (5)

Globally, of the 300 million adolescent women, approximately 16 million give birth each year, representing one in ten of all births. Adolescent pregnancy is a global health and social problem. In 2015, according to the World Health Organization (WHO), 303,000 maternal deaths occurred worldwide, of which 7,900 were in the Americas, where the adolescent mother contributes considerably to this mortality, which is influenced by the region where she lives; in a 15-year-old adolescent the mortality rate is 1 in 4,900 in developed countries, and 1 in 180 in developing countries. The adolescent fertility rate among 10-14 year olds was 1.5 births per 1 000 girls/adolescents, which means between 6 and 7 births per day (WHO, 2018). Of European countries, England has the highest incidence, around 9 000 adolescents become pregnant, while in Spain there are 18 000 pregnancies per year in this age group.(4, 6, 7)

Latin America and the Caribbean is one of the regions where births to girls under the age of 15 are on the rise and are expected to continue to increase slightly until 2030. In 2015, there were 107 million girls and adolescents in the Latin America and Caribbean region, which corresponds to 17 per cent of the region's total population. Brazil has the largest population of girls and adolescents, followed by Mexico and Colombia. Two million children are born each year to mothers aged 15-19 in Latin America and the Caribbean. This is the second region in the world with the highest specific fertility rate, 61 per 1 000 women aged 15-19 (2015-2020), preceded by 109 per 1 000 in Sub-Saharan Africa.(8, 9)

The most significant countries in the Americas are Colombia (2017) with a fertility rate of 61.11; Argentina, with 53.1; and Costa Rica (2018), with a fertility rate of 48.3 (5, 10).

Looking at Cuba in particular (2019), the population in the adolescent stage is close to more than 1.5 million people, or almost 11 %. During 2019, the fertility rate for women aged 15-19 was 52.3 per 1,000 women, and in Villa Clara it was 52 per 1,000 women. In the municipality of Ranchuelo, Villa Clara, at the end of 2018, the number of pregnant adolescents who gave birth was 40. According to the Department of Municipal Statistics, 110 underwent termination of pregnancy, including curettage and regulation.(11)

Cuba carries out actions with the aim of preventing teenage pregnancy, an example of this is the intervention study carried out in the Capitán Silverio Blanco Núñez Urban Basic Secondary School, in the municipality of Camagüey, in the period from October 2015 to February 2016. There, once the learning needs had been identified, a system of educational actions was designed and subsequently evaluated. Before applying the educational intervention, it was found that the adolescents did not have adequate knowledge about how to prevent pregnancy at this age; after the actions were carried out, it was found that this knowledge improved· Another example is the educational intervention carried out in Clinic # 17, Guillermo González Polanco Polyclinic, in Guisa, from June 2016 to January 2017, where knowledge was successfully modified (12, 13).

During the period from January to June 2018 in the municipality of El Salvador, Guantánamo, an educational intervention with community participation was carried out in the Reynaldo Castro complex. Before the intervention, adolescent girls had a low level of knowledge. After the intervention, knowledge was raised in relation to contraceptive use, optimal age for pregnancy, the main risks and complications of abortion, for an overall level of knowledge of good. (14)

Pregnancy at an early age is currently a major challenge. The consequences of this problem have repercussions on the quality of life of the young mother and her family, and pose a significant risk to her offspring. The community is not exempt from this conflict, and is in some way involved in the outcome of this dramatic event.(14)

Adolescents are a high-risk group, as their advanced sexual maturation leads them to seek early sexual relations. This exposes them to sexually transmitted infections and early pregnancy, which usually occurs due to lack of contraceptive use, and they are inadequately prepared for sexual relations. Complex biological, psychological and social changes are now considered to occur at this stage of life, making it increasingly necessary to devote attention to it.

Adolescent pregnancy is a social, economic, educational and psychological conflict problem of considerable magnitude, both for young people and for their children, partners, family, community and institutions such as Public Health and Education. It is one of the main factors contributing to maternal and infant mortality, psychological disorders, among others. The family doctor, within the framework of public health in Cuba, plays an important role in the care of adolescents, as well as contributing to fostering timely social behaviour in adolescents and providing attention to the physical, emotional and social aspects that form the personality.(15)

In the Mario Muñoz Monroy polyclinic, in the town of Esperanza and belonging to the municipality of Ranchuelo, there were a total of 70 teenage pregnancies in 2018, of which 61 underwent some type of pregnancy termination and 9 reached full term.

In the health area corresponding to the Family Medical Clinic (CMF) #5 of the Mario Muñoz Monroy Polyclinic, in recent years there has been an increase in pregnancies at this stage due to the fact that the majority of adolescents do not protect themselves with any contraceptive method, are not controlled as a preconceptional risk, consume alcohol, as well as a deficient level of information on the adequate control of modifiable risk factors. In addition, it has been found that the risk factors that cause this problem are not controlled by health personnel. So far this year, 19 adolescents have become pregnant and 16 of these have undergone some method of pregnancy termination, including menstrual regulation. This situation is worrying both for the clinic and for the corresponding health area, where there are adolescents who have already gestated more than once, hence the motivation for carrying out this research, and the following **scientific problem** is posed:

How to improve the control of modifiable risk factors associated with adolescent pregnancy in CMF # 5 of Esperanza from February 2020 to February 2022?

Hypothesis: An educational programme for adolescents belonging to the Medical Clinic #5 of the Mario Muñoz Monroy polyclinic in the town of Esperanza will make it possible to control modifiable risk factors associated with adolescent pregnancy, such as: improving the level of information, family functioning, control of preconceptional reproductive risk, reducing alcohol consumption, increasing the use of condoms and other contraceptive methods, maintaining continuity of studies and reducing the occurrence of sexually transmitted diseases, as well as reducing the incidence of pregnancy in the adolescents studied in the period February 2020-February 2022.

2 OBJECTIVES

GENERAL OBJECTIVE:

- To determine the effectiveness of an educational programme for adolescents to control modifiable risk factors associated with adolescent pregnancy at the Esperanza Medical Clinic #5 in the period February 2020-February 2022.

SPECIFIC OBJECTIVES:

- Characterise the sample according to epidemiological and social variables.
- To determine the level of knowledge about adolescent pregnancy before and after the education programme.
- To establish the relationship between the implementation of the educational programme and the control of modifiable risk factors associated with adolescent pregnancy in the patients studied.

3 THEORETICAL FRAMEWORK

Adolescence is defined as the period of life between the ages of 10 and 19· It is a stage of transition towards adulthood, of adaptation to social and economic independence and includes the development of identity. For some authors, it is the phase in which the child becomes an adult, and where physical and psychological changes take place at an accelerated pace. Among the most important biological changes are: the onset of menstruation in girls, the presence of sperm in boys, the maturation of the reproductive organs and the attainment of sexual maturity (6, 16-19).

In accordance with the above, it will be pertinent, firstly, to normalise adolescence; that is, among other things, to recognise its characteristics, free adolescents from stereotypes and prejudices, be empathetic and understanding, yet demanding and capable of containing them. And, secondly, to assume the responsibility we have as adults to accompany and guide the formative and developmental processes of adolescents, in a world in which science and various disciplines have made it possible to understand the needs and risks of this stage of the life cycle. In this way, we can contribute to the development of mentally healthy adults(20).

The stages of adolescence are: early, middle and late adolescence.

Early adolescence (between 10 and 14 years of age)

During this stage, children often begin to grow faster. They also begin to notice other body changes, including the growth of hair in the armpits and genital area, and breast development in females. It usually begins one to two years earlier in girls than in boys, and it may be normal for some changes to begin as early as age 8 for girls and age 9 for boys. Many girls have their first menstruation around the age of 12, on average 2 to 3 years after the start of breast development.(18, 19)

These bodily changes may generate curiosity and anxiety for some, especially if they do not know what to expect or what is normal. Some children also question their gender identity at this stage, and the onset of puberty can be a difficult time for transgender children (18, 19).

Younger teenagers have concrete and extremist ideas. Things are either right or wrong, fantastic or terrible, without much nuance. At this stage it is normal for young people to focus their thinking on themselves (what we call 'egocentrism'). As part of this, pre-teens and younger adolescents often feel self-conscious about their appearance and feel as if they are constantly being judged by their peers.(18, 19)

Pre-teens have an increased need for privacy. They may begin to explore ways to be independent from their family. In this process, they are likely to test boundaries and react strongly if parents or guardians assert limits.

Middle adolescence (15-16 years)

Physical changes that began at puberty continue through middle adolescence. Most boys begin their "growth spurt" and puberty-related changes continue. They may, for example, have a cracking voice as they get older. Some may develop acne. Physical changes are likely to be almost complete in females, and most girls already have regular menses.(18, 19)

At this age, many adolescents become interested in romantic and sexual relationships. They may be questioning and exploring their sexual identity, which can be stressful if they do not have the support of their peers, family or community.(18, 19)

Another typical way for adolescents of all genders to explore sex and sexuality is self-stimulation, also called masturbation.

Many young people in their mid-teens argue more with their parents because they struggle to have more independence. They are likely to spend less time with family and more time with friends. They are very concerned about their appearance and peer pressure can peak at this stage. The brain is still changing and maturing at this stage, but there are still many differences between the thinking of a young person in their mid-teens and an adult. Much of this is because the frontal lobes are the last area of the brain to mature; development is not complete until a person is in their early twenties. The frontal lobes play an important role in coordinating complex decision-making, impulse control and the ability to consider various options and consequences. Young people in their mid-teens are better able to think abstractly and keep the "big picture" in mind, but still lack the ability to apply it in the moment. (18)

Late adolescence (17-19 years)

Young people in late adolescence have usually completed physical development and have reached the final height they will have as adults. By this age they tend to have more control over their impulses and can weigh risks and rewards better and more accurately.

Adolescents who become young adults now have a stronger sense of their own individuality and can identify their own values. They are more focused on the future and base their decisions on their illusions and ideals. Friendships and romantic relationships become more stable. They separate more from their family, both physically and emotionally. However, many re-establish an "adult" relationship with their parents, seeing them as peers to ask for advice and talk to about serious issues, rather than as an authority figure. (18)

The **adolescent** stage of the life cycle is characterised by increased psychosocial vulnerability, an increased need to regulate affect and behaviour through self-goals that are often different from those goals provided by adults during childhood (Steinberg, 2005, 2007). Increased adolescent risk-taking has been explained by the fragile balance between sensation-seeking and novelty, especially from early **adolescence** onwards, and the capacity for self-regulation, which is still immature and does not fully develop until the early teenage years (Steinberg, 2005).

Globally, adolescent pregnancy continues to be an impediment to improving the educational, economic and social status of women.(21, 22)

It is a major health problem recognised by the World Health Organisation (WHO) and the international community, exemplified by the alarming statistics published worldwide:(21)

- The global adolescent pregnancy rate is estimated at 46 births per 1,000 girls, while adolescent pregnancy rates in Latin America and the Caribbean remain the second highest in the world, estimated at 66.5 births per 1,000 girls aged 15-19.
- Some 16 million girls aged 15-19 and approximately 1 million girls under 15 give birth each year.
- Complications during pregnancy and childbirth are the second leading cause of death among girls aged 15-19 worldwide.
- Babies born to teenage mothers face a significantly higher risk of dying than those born to women aged 20-24.
- Although there has been a significant, albeit uneven, decline in adolescent birth rates over the past three decades, approximately 11 per cent of all births worldwide are still to girls aged 15-19. The vast majority of these births (95 per cent) occur in low- and middle-income countries.
- The number of births to teenage mothers rises to 16 million each year globally
- Currently, the world's population is estimated at 6090 million, 17.5 % are individuals between 10-19 years of age; of these, 10 % become pregnant, which is equivalent to 10 % of all births worldwide. This means that approximately 16 million women aged 10-19 years have a birth every year.(21)

Adolescent pregnancy is a global phenomenon with clearly known causes and serious health, social and economic consequences for the individuals concerned, their families and communities. There is consensus on the evidence-based actions needed to prevent it. There is growing global, regional and national commitment to prevent child marriage and adolescent pregnancy and childbearing. Non-governmental organizations have been at the forefront of the fight in a number of countries. In an increasing number of countries, governments are taking the lead in launching large-scale programmes.(1)

Studies of risk and protective factors related to adolescent pregnancy in lower middle-income countries indicate that levels tend to be higher among those with less education or low economic status. Progress in reducing adolescent first births has been particularly slow among these vulnerable groups, which has led to growing inequality.(1, 7)

Factors influencing the number of adolescent pregnancies and births(1).

- In many societies, girls are pressured to marry and have children. In the year 2021, the estimated number of child brides in the world was 650 million. In many places, girls choose to become pregnant because their educational and employment prospects are poor.

- In many places, adolescents do not have easy access to contraceptive methods. Even when they can obtain them, they may lack the means or resources to pay for them, as well as the knowledge of where to obtain them and how to use them correctly.
- Restrictive laws and policies regarding the provision of contraceptives based on age or marital status are a major barrier to contraceptive provision and uptake among adolescents. (7)
- Often, this is combined with the prejudice or unwillingness of health personnel to recognise the sexual health needs of adolescents.
- By 2020, it is estimated that at least 1 in 8 children worldwide will have experienced sexual abuse by the age of 18, and 1 in 20 girls aged 15-19 will have experienced forced sex in their lifetime(1, 7).

METHODOLOGY

A quasi-experimental longitudinal intervention study was carried out without a control group, prospectively in the Family Medical Clinic #5 of the Mario Muñoz Monroy polyclinic in the village of Esperanza, belonging to the municipality of Ranchuelo, in the period from February 2020-February 2022.

The population consisted of 35 female adolescents.

The sample consisted of 24 adolescents, 68.6% of the population, drawn intentionally (non-probabilistic), who met the inclusion and exclusion criteria.

Inclusion Criteria:

J Willingness to participate in the research after the importance of the research has been explained to them (Informed Consent Annex 1).

J Consent of parents or legal guardian (Annex 2).

J Female adolescents from the medical clinic #5 of the Mario Muñoz Monroy polyclinic in the village of Esperanza, municipality of Ranchuelo, who were in the area during the study period.

J Be physically and mentally fit to participate in the study.

J Not having been involved in any other influence related to the subject.

Exclusion Criteria

J Adolescents unwilling to participate in the study.

J Adolescents who are out of the area in the study period.

J Failure to answer all the questions in the diagnostic instruments.

J - Participate in less than 10 group activities.

Different methods, both theoretical and empirical, were applied.

1. Theoretical level methods:

Historical-logical method: The historical method allowed the study of the real trajectory of the phenomena and events in the course of their history and the logical method allowed the general laws of the functioning and development of the investigative phenomena to be known.

Analytical-synthetic method: This was used for the systematisation of the bibliographical study and the interpretation of the results of the empirical methods.

Inductive-deductive method: Inductive and deductive reasoning, starting from the formulation of a hypothesis.

Abstract-concrete method: It allowed finding associations between variables.

2. Empirical level methods:

Experiment: Quasi-experimental type. Where measurements are taken before and after the educational intervention is carried out.

Documentary review: Through the review of medical records and archived epidemiological surveys, modifiable risk factors associated with adolescent pregnancy were identified, and information was collected using a model developed for this purpose.

Survey: In order to obtain the information, a survey was applied to collect the variables of interest, the epidemiological variables (Annex # 3).

In addition, a questionnaire to determine the needs in terms of the level of information on the topic for the intervention, before and after the educational programme was implemented. Annex 4.

The study consisted of three phases:

First phase: Educational Planning and Diagnosis.

In this phase, the adolescents included in the study were characterised and the needs for intervention were determined, and the main risk factors related to the health problem to be investigated were also identified by means of a survey (Appendix #3). In addition, a documentary review of the Family Health History (HSF) and Individual Clinical History was carried out, which allowed for the identification of modifiable and non-modifiable risk factors, as well as the characterisation of the study group by means of the variables. Visits were made to the families of the adolescents participating in the study, where family functioning was assessed according to the dynamics of internal family relationships by applying the FF-SIL test (Appendix 4).

A questionnaire was applied (Annex 5) with selection questions to measure the knowledge that adolescents have about the topic to be investigated. The questions were adapted to the thematic content and objectives of the workshops, and were enriched by consulting questionnaires reported in national and international literature. The questionnaire is worth 100 points and each item was rated depending on the content of the questionnaire. Each aspect of the content was analysed and those who did not reach 70 % of the total score of the test were assessed as insufficient. The knowledge test was filled out individually by each adolescent. The initial cut-off was made at the first meeting. From this point onwards, the educational intervention began, and the final one in the second phase of the research.

Second phase: Implementation.

Based on the risk factors and learning needs identified through the application of the questionnaire (Annex 5), an educational programme was designed that covered aspects related to modifiable risk factors associated with adolescent pregnancy (Annex 6).

At this stage, 11 meetings were held, each lasting 60 minutes. Over a period of 12 months. The sample was divided into two groups to be taught in a monthly session, using different participatory techniques. The topics were dedicated to the different sections corresponding to each question of the previously applied test.

The main themes of the educational programme were reinforced through family visits. To this end, the frequency of these visits was increased and the participation of all family members present was encouraged. The evaluations of each activity with the group were recorded in the HSF.

In addition, the adolescents underwent monthly check-ups and a monthly field visit every four months, where they underwent exhaustive questioning and a complete physical examination, and a contraceptive method was negotiated with the sexually active adolescent, as well as interconsultations with gynaecology and obstetrics, consultations with these adolescents in order to evaluate the control of modifiable risk factors, and interconsultations with psychology, when necessary, and gynaecobstetrics. Visits were made to the family every two months in order to carry out family counselling: a communication process through which the basic health team helped the family to identify their health needs and suggested alternative solutions. Families were consulted by the psychologist in the area.

Third phase: Evaluation

To assess the level of knowledge acquired, the same initial questionnaire (Annex 5) was used to obtain results on the study variables. When compared with the initial results, the modification of modifiable risk factors was evaluated, based on the risk controls.

Data processing and analysis assessed whether modifiable risk factors such as contraceptive use, especially condom use, alcohol consumption associated with sexual intercourse, and increased levels of information were controlled for.

In this phase, the success of the programme was assessed on the basis of the achievements of the last questionnaire and knowledge test. It will be determined whether the objectives of the programme were achieved, thus completing the third stage.

Operationalisation of variables

Dimensions	Variables	Type of variable	Description	Measurement scale
Risks No modifi cables	Stages of adolescence.	la Quantitativ a Continuous.	Adolescent's age since date of birth at baseline.	Adolescence '/ Early (between 10 and 14 years) '/ Intermediate (between 15 and 16 years) '/ Late (between 17 and 19 years).
	Schooling.	Qualitative Ordinal.	According to the last level completed.	'/ Primary. '/ Secondary. '/ Pre-university.
Dimensions	**Variables**	**Type of variable**	**Description**	**Measuring scale**
sexual	Age of first relations	the Quantitativ a continua.	Years attained by the adolescent in the time when she had her first intercourse.	'/ Under 12 years of age '/ between 12-14 years old '/ more than 15 years.
Type of link of a couple		Qualitative Nominal Politomica.	Particularities of the couple's relationship.	'/ Boyfriend '/ Married '/ Concubinage
Background on abortions provoked		Qualitative nominal dichotomous	Obstetric history related to la presence of voluntary interruptions of gestation.	J Yes J No
Dimensions Variables		**Type of variable**	**Description**	**Measuring scale**

Cause realisation from induced abortion from	Qualitative Nominal Politomica.	Reason(s) for requesting the abortion.	What the patient refers to, by For example: age, other young children, partner pressure, family pressure, interruption of personal development, financial difficulties or housing difficulties.

Dimensions Variables	Type of Description Measuring scale variable
Background relatives of pregnancy in the adolescence	Grandmother(s): J YES J NO Mother: Question on the background of v' YES Qualitative adolescent pregnancy in J NO nominal Next of kin: Aunt(s): polytomics J Yes v' No Sister(s): J Yes J No

Dimensions Variables	Type of DescriptionMeasuring scale variable
Types from infections of Riskstransmission modificadlessexual (STI)diagnostics das.	J HIV-AIDS. '/ Blennorrhagia. Infections that are transmittedSyphilis . Qualitative mainly due to the relationships Trichomonas. Nominal sexual and some of them by contact Chlamydia. Politomica. with infected blood from the mother to her hepatitis B and C. son. J Herpes Simplex. '/ Condyloma.

'/ Unknown.

Dimensions	Variables	Type of variable	Description	Measurement scale
	Operation Family.	Qualitative ordinal	Family functionability refers to to the relatively stable characteristic the group's internal relations. It is the set of relationships interpersonal relationships that are established in the within each family and which give them identity, before and after applied the programme According to the test called FF-SIL (Annex 2).	Family Functional from 70 to 57 points. '/ Moderately Functional from 56 to 43 points. '/ Dysfunctional from 42 to 28 points. '/ Severely Dysfunctional from 27 to 14 points.

	All methods will be taken into account	'/ Condom.
	contraceptives that are marketed and	J D.I.U (T for copper, multiload, handle,
	recommended by practitioners.	
Types	from	
	Qualitative Contraceptive: instruments or	Tablets.
methods		
	Nominal Substances that prevent the	'/ Rhythm method.
contraceptives		
	Polytomy. fertilisation or nesting in the	'/ Coitus interruptus.
which uses		'/ Surgical
	uterine cavity, before and after	
		'/ Unknown.
	implemented the programme, before and	
implemented the programme		

Dimensions Variables Type of

Variable description

Measurement scale

Never

Qualitative The consumption of alcoholic beverages, prior to

'/ Sometimes alcohol. ordinal and after the programme has been applied

'/ Almost always

Dimensions Variables	**Type of variable**	**Description**	**Measurement scale**
Risk control reproductive preconception	Qualitative nominal dichotomous	It is the periodic assessment of women with RRPC, the frequency of which will depend on risk and severity, with the aim of achieving risk mitigation with the as quickly as possible. It includes guidance on the availability of contraceptive methods, safe and effective as long as the risk is mitigated or eliminated.	'/ Controlled: This is when 1 consultation, 1 ground per year EBS is carried out. '/ Uncontrolled: This is when 1 enquiry was not made o 1 plot for the EBS annual.

Dimensions	**Variables**	**Type of variable**	**Description**	**Measuring scale**

Level information about pregnancy in adolescence.	from Qualitative on Ordinal la	Adolescent girls' level of preparedness on teenage pregnancy according to the score obtained in the questionnaire before and after the implementation of the educational programme.	Good: 80 points and above. Rθgular' 70 to 79 points en e Wrong: 69 points or less. of la

Data collection

Several techniques were used to collect the information: the structured interview, which was applied to each adolescent individually and was designed to obtain information on socio-demographic characteristics; a survey to answer the research objectives. (Annex 2).

The form collected data of interest on modifiable and non-modifiable epidemiological factors, which were deposited in a computerised database using Excel, then imported from IBM SPSS Statistic Version 25 for statistical processing.

Analysis techniques will be used according to the study design. For the interpretation of the results we will determine the mean between ages. Frequency and contingency tables were constructed to analyse the relationship between variables.

The following hypothesis tests were used from inferential statistics:

Chi-square of independence to determine the relationship between two variables or differences between the categories of one variable with respect to the other.

Chi-square goodness-of-fit to determine differences between categories of a variable.

Binomial test to determine differences between categories of a dichotomous variable.

Sign test (ordinal variables) to determine significant changes in a qualitative, polytomous variable before and after applying a system of influences.

Homogeneity test (categorical variables) marginal to determine significant changes in a qualitative, polytomous variable before and after applying a system of influences.

In order to make a decision, the significance levels of 0.1, 0.05 and 0.01 were compared with the significance of the test (p), making the decision as follows:

If $p<0.01$: There is a highly significant relationship, difference or change.

If $p<0.05$ Significant relationship, differences or changes exist

If p<0.1: There is a moderately significant relationship, difference or change.

If p≥0.1 No significant relationship, difference or change

Ethical considerations: The work was carried out with the aim of providing elements that contribute to improving human health, in compliance with the principles of Bioethics. Informed consent was given to patients and their guardians as they were adolescents (Annex 1 and 2), and to the Ethics Committee of the research. On the other hand, the information obtained will be confidential and for scientific use.

RESULTS

Table 1. Distribution of adolescent patients according to stage of adolescence and schooling at the Family Medical Clinic #5 of the Mario Muñoz Monroy polyclinic in the village of Esperanza, belonging to the municipality of Ranchuelo, in the period February 2020-February 2022.

Schooling

T Stage[otal]

Secondary Pre-university

adolescence

	No.	%	No.	%	No.	%
Early	3	100	0	0	3	12,5
Intermediate	2	25	6	75	8	33,3
Late	0	0	13	100		1354,2
Total	5	20,8	19	79,2		24100,0

Survey source.

Chi-square Goodness of fit. Adolescence stage χ^2 =6.250; p=0.044

Chi-square Goodness of fit. Schooling χ^2 =8.1; p=0.004.

Chi-square of independence χ^2 =14.905; p=0.000

As can be seen in table 1. There is a significant predominance (χ^2 =6.250; p=0.044) of patients in late adolescence, 54.2%, and a very significant predominance (χ^2 =8.1; p=0.004) of adolescents with pre-university level, 19 patients representing 79.2%. Overall, there is a highly significant relationship (χ^2 =14.905; p=0.000) between the variables schooling and stage of adolescence, with late adolescents predominating in Pre-university and middle-stage adolescents in Secondary.

Table 2. Distribution of patients with respect to age at first intercourse and type of partner relationship.

Age	Type of partnership						Total	
First sexual	Married		Concubinage		Boyfriend			
intercourse	No.	%	No.	%	No.	%	No.	%
13 years	0	0,0	0	0,0	4	100	4	16,7
14 years	0	0.0	4	57,1	3	42,9	7	29,2

15 years	2	18,2	3	27,3	6	54,5	11	45,8
16 years	1	50,2	0	0,0	1	50,0	2	8,3
Total	3	12,5	7	29,2	14	58,3	24	100,0

Source: Survey

Chi-square Goodness of fit. Age of first relationships χ^2 =16.667; p=0.000

Chi-square Goodness of fit. Relationship type χ^2 =7.750 p=0.021

Chi-square of independence χ^2 =9.08; p=0.169.

Table 2 shows a significant predominance (χ^2 =7.750 p=0.021) of adolescent girls with a boyfriend relationship, 14 patients for 58.3%. And a predominance of girls with first sexual intercourse at 15 years of age, 11 patients (45.8%).

There is no significant relationship between the age of first sexual relations and the type of partnership, as the distributions of patients by age of first sexual relations with respect to the types of partnership do not differ, only those who started their sexual relations at 14 years of age, the highest percentage corresponds to those who are cohabiting.

Table 3. Distribution of patients according to cause of miscarriage

Causes	Abortions	
	YES	NO
Age	3	0
No answer	0	14
Family Pressure	3	0
Economic difficulties	4	0
Total	10	14

Source: Survey

p*Significance binomial test: Abortion (Yes, No) p=0.541

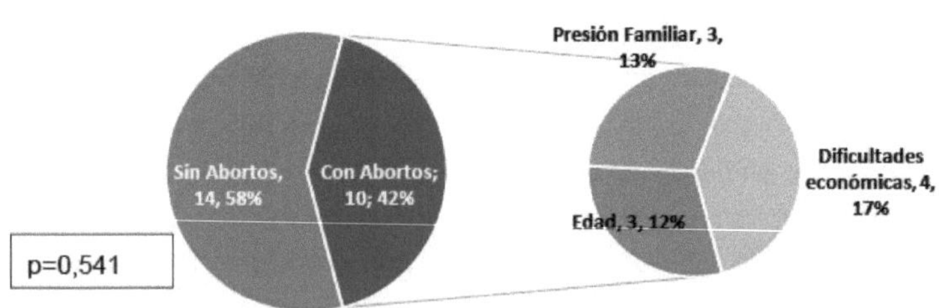

Graph 1. Distribution of patients according to abortions and causes of abortion

Source Table 1.

As shown in Table 3, Figure 1, there is no significant difference between the proportion of patients who report not having abortions and those who do, and the predominant cause of forced abortions is economic hardship.

Table 4. Distribution of patients according to family history of adolescent pregnancy.

Family	No.	%
Mother	5	20,8
Aunt	2	8,3
Sisters	4	16,7
No family history	13	54,1

Survey source.

Chi-square test for goodness-of-fit family background χ^2 =11.667; p=0.009

According to table 4, the absence of a family history of teenage pregnancy is highly significant (χ^2 =11.667; p=0.009), 13 patients, 54.1%. The highest percentage of patients with a history of adolescent pregnancy corresponds to the maternal branch (20.8%).

Table 5. Distribution of the patients according to sexually transmitted infections suffered

ITS	No.	%	p
Blenpragia	1	4,2	0,000
Herpes simpli	2	8,3	0,000
Chlamydia	2	8,3	0,000
Condyloma	1	4,2	0,000
Total	6	25,0	0,000

Survey source.

p: significance of the binomial test

Table 5 shows that the absence of sexually transmitted infections in the patients is significant: only 6 patients, 25%, have sexually transmitted infections, and of these, herpes simpli and chlamydia are the most frequent.

Table 6. Distribution of patients according to alcohol consumption before and after the educational programme.

Alcohol consumption After								
Consumption of alcohol Before	Never		Sometimes		Most of the time		Total	
	No.	%	No.	%	No.	%	No.	%
Never	13	100,0	0	0,0	0	0,0	13	54,2
Sometimes	1	16,7	5	83,3	0	0,0	6	25,0
Most of the time	0	0,0	1	33,3	2	66,7	3	12,5
Always	0	0,0	0	0,0	2	100,0	2	8,3
Total	14	58,3	6	25	4	16,7	24	100,0

Survey source.

Sign test (binomial distribution used): p=0.125 4 patients decrease, 20 no change

As can be seen in table 6, before applying the educational programme, there is a predominance of those who never consume alcohol 13 patients, 54.2%, followed by those who consume alcohol sometimes, 25%, and after applying the programme, the predominance of those who never consume alcohol is maintained, 58%, followed by those who consume alcohol sometimes. 58%, followed by those who drink sometimes. The 13 patients who did not consume alcohol remained without consuming it, of the 6 patients who consumed it sometimes, 5 remained and one of them stopped consuming alcohol, and the two who always consumed alcohol went on to consume it almost always. Although the change in alcohol consumption is not significant, there was a decrease in alcohol consumption.

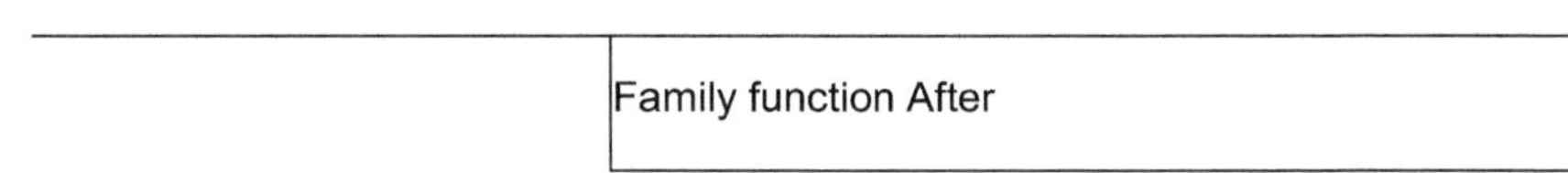
Family function After

Table 7. Distribution of patients according to family function Before and after the educational programme was applied

Functional

Family function Before	Moderately Functional				Total	
	No.	%	No.	%	No.	%
Dysfunctional Family	1	100	0	0	1	4,2
Moderately Functional	6	85,7	1	14,3	7	29,2
Functional Family	0	0	16	100	16	66,7
Total	7	29,2	17	70,8	24	100,0

Survey source.

Sign test p=0.5. The binomial distribution was used

As can be seen in table 7, before the educational programme was applied, there was a significant predominance of functional families 16 patients, 67%, followed by moderately functional families, a predominance that was maintained after the educational programme was applied. Although there are no significant differences with the change, an improvement is observed, highlighting the absence of dysfunctional families and an increase in functional families.

Table 8. Distribution of patients according to contraceptive method before and after the educational programme was implemented.

Contraceptives	Contraceptives After	Total

Formerly	Tablet		Condom		None			
	No.	%	No.	%	No.	%	No.	%
Tablet	3	100	0	0	0	0	3	12,5
Condom	0	0	10	100	0		010	41,7
Coitus interruptus	2	33,3	4	66,7	0	0	6	25,0
None	3	60	1	20	1	20	5	20,8
Total	8	33,3	15	62,5	1	4,2	24	100,0

Survey source.

Marginal Homogeneity Test: HM=34; p=0.004

As can be seen in table 8, the change in the use of contraceptives by the patients is very significant (: HM=34; p=0.004); in which the 5 who did not use contraceptives, only one patient remains, of the 6 who used coitus interruptus, two of them use tablets and 4 use condoms after the programme was applied.

Table 9. Distribution of patients according to preconception reproductive risk control.

Preconception reproductive risk management.	No.	%
YES	18	75,0
NO	6	25,0

Survey source.

Significance of the binomial test: p=0,023

As shown in table 9, 75% of the patients were subjected to reproductive risk monitoring.

Table. 10 Level of information before and after the educational programme was implemented.

Level of information before	Level of information after				Total	
	Regular		Well			
	No.	%	No.	%	No.	%
Mal	2	66,7	1	33,3	3	12,5
Regular	3	25	9	75	12	50,0
Well	0	0	9	100	9	37,5
Total	5	20,8	19	79,2	24	100,0

Source: Knowledge test

Sign test: p=0.000

As can be seen in table 10, before the educational programme was applied, there was a predominance of patients with a fair level of information; after the programme was applied, there were very significant changes ($p<0.01$), with a predominance of patients with a good level of information and no patients with a poor level of information.

4 DISCUSSION OF THE RESULTS

The study consists of an educational programme for the control of modifiable risk factors associated with adolescent pregnancy, in which the risk factors associated with adolescent pregnancy are analysed. Since there are not many studies that refer to educational programmes, those studies that allow us to describe the present variables are analysed.

Table 1. Distribution of adolescent patients according to stage of adolescence and schooling at the Family Medical Clinic #5 of the Mario Muñoz Monroy polyclinic in the village of Esperanza, belonging to the municipality of Ranchuelo, in the period February 2020-February 2022.

In studies carried out by Mazuera and colleagues(23) in Venezuela, with a sample of adolescents between 10 and 19 years of age, in the State of Táchira, patients between 17 and 19 years of age predominated, similar to the distribution of the stages of adolescence in the present study, with 86.1% at secondary school level, the lowest school level.

According to studies carried out by Jacome-Gallegos et al (24) and collaborators, 52% of pregnant adolescents belong to the 17-19 age group; 33% correspond to the 14-16 age group, while 15% of women are 10-13 years old, similar to the present study. The mothers' level of schooling reflects 45% primary school, while 40% high school, the lowest level of schooling (24).

Table 2. shows that there is a predominance of teenage girls who live together as boyfriends and girlfriends, which is very common nowadays, corresponding to teenage girls aged 13 years old.

In the study carried out by Mazuera and collaborators(23) there is a predominance of those who are called united, in Cuba, they are called concubinage, or consensual union, 53.19%.

Alava Mariscal, 90% of pregnant adolescents began having sexual relations between 15 and 16 years of age, coinciding with this work(25).

Jacome-Gallegos et al. (24) 25% of adolescent girls have initiated their sexual life before the age of 20, a coinciding element.

Table 3. and Graph 1. In the present study 42% of pregnant women have resorted to abortion and the predominant cause of forced abortions is economic hardship.

Table 4.

Table 4 of the present study shows the distribution of patients according to family history of adolescent pregnancy in which 54.1% did not have a family history. Similar results were found in the study by González (26).

Table 5.

Distribution of patients according to sexually transmitted infections suffered, where Herpes simpli and chlamydia are the most frequent. In a study carried out by Ferrer Santos (27), 29.3% had Trichomoniasis, 24.4% Chlamydia, 15.9% Gardnerella,

14.6% Gonorrhoea, 11.0% and 4.9% Syphilis, with the results coinciding only in the presence of Chlamydia.

Table 6 shows the distribution of patients according to alcohol consumption, with a predominance of those who never drink alcohol Jacome-Gallegos et al. have similar results to the present study (24).

Table 7. In the present study, there is a predominance of functional families, which does not coincide with studies carried out by Jacome-Gallegos and collaborators, more than half belong to dysfunctional families (24),

Table 8 shows that there was a significant change in the use of contraceptive methods, coinciding with the studies of Cos Hernández and collaborators(28) in an educational intervention to modify criteria on early pregnancy and its risks among adolescents in the Reynaldo Castro complex in the municipality of El Salvador. In Guantánamo, only 84.6% used some contraceptive method and after the intervention, all of them did so, positively changing their behaviour(28).

Table 9. In this study, 75% of the patients were subjected to reproductive risk control. Similar results are found in Zetina(29). A high percentage of the women in this study were at a medium preconception risk level, which could lead to a future pregnancy with obstetric complications that could put the mother and foetus at risk.

Table 10. Level of information before and after the educational programme was applied, a very significant change is obtained in the change of information levels, in favour of the increase, similar results obtained by Cos Hernández and collaborators (28).

This demonstrates the effectiveness of the educational programme for the control of modifiable risk factors associated with adolescent pregnancy in CMF#5. Esperanza .

5 CONCLUSIONS

There is a significant predominance of patients in late adolescence, with pre-university level, first sexual relations at 15 years of age and cohabitation, the cause of forced abortions is economic difficulties, no family history of teenage pregnancies, no sexually transmitted infections, the following factors were modified: alcohol consumption, family function, use of contraceptives.

There is a very significant change in the level of information in a positive way.

6 BIBLIOGRAPHICAL REFERENCES

1. OMdl Health, Td Health. Adolescent pregnancy. 2022 [Available fro m : https://www.who.int/es/news-room/fact-sheets/detail/adolescent-pregnancy#.
2. Ley Vega L VRT, Satorre Ygualada JA, Satorre Ygualada S, García Alemán A, Satorre Ley MK. . Adolescent pregnancy and cardiovascular risk factors . Acta Médica del Centro [Internet] 2019 13(2).
3. WHO. Adolescent Pregnancy. 2022.
4. Figueroa Verdecia D, Navarro Sánchez Y, Romero Guzmán F. Current situation of adolescence and its main challenges . Gac med espirit [Internet].
2018 20.(1):approx.6p.
5. Medina O, Ortiz K. Adolescent fertility and social inequalities in Mexico, 2015. Rev Panam Salud Publica 4230 2018; 43(5).
6. Mejia C, Delgado M, Mostto F, Torres R, Díaz A, Cárdenas M, et al. Abuse during adolescent pregnancy: A descriptive study in pregnant women attending a public hospital in Lima. Revista chilena de obstetricia y ginecología 2018;83 (1): approx. 5 p.
7. Health. OPdl. Adolescent Pregnancy in Latin America and the Caribbean Technical Review 2020.
8. Póo M, Aravena G, Mieres Y, Canales P. Meaning given to parenthood during pregnancy by adolescent parents. . Index Enferm [Internet] 2018;27(3).
9. Restrepo AM, Muñoz Y, Duque MA. Analysis of the elements of social marketing implicit in adolescent pregnancy prevention campaigns. Revista Facultad Nacional de Salud Pública, [Internet]. 2018 36(2).
10. Ortiz Martínez R, Otalora Perdomo M, Delgado M, Luna D. Adolescence as a risk factor for maternal and neonatal complications. Revista chilena de obstetricia y ginecología [Internet] 2018; 83(5):478-86.
11. Public. MoH. Health Statistical Yearbook 2019. Havana. In: Salud DNdRMyEd, editor. Habana2020.
12. Figueredo M, Aguilar S, Vinajera A. Educational intervention on adolescent pregnancy in CMF 17, Guisa June 2016-January 2017. Nursing Journal. 2017;23(4).
13. Olivera CC BA, Sotolongo IM. Educational intervention to prevent adolescent pregnancy. . Technosalud 2016; 19 (3).
14. Hernández C, Brooks Salazar Y, Salgado Rodríguez M. Educational intervention on adolescent pregnancy in the Reynaldo Castro complex. El Salvador . Nursing journal
2019.;8(3).
15. Taily RB, Lya del Rosario MA, Laura Mary SP, Maira QE, editors. GLOBAL ADOLESCENT PREGNANCY ANALYSIS.
UPDATE. cibamanz2021; 2021.
16. Bulgach V, Zunana C, Califano P, Rodríguez MS, Mato R. Adolescent mothers

hospitalized with their children in a high complexity hospital: differences between early-mid and late adolescence. Arch argent pediatr. 2018;116(2):160-4.
17. Vilela M, Sandoval Ato R, Galvez Olortegui J. Prevention and support strategies in adolescents with depression and suicidal behaviour: an urgent need. . Cuban Journal of General Comprehensive Medicine [Internet]. 2018 33 (4).
18. Brittany Allen M, FAAP and Helen Waterman D. Stages of adolescence. Helthy childrenor in English
19. Allen B, Waterman H. Stages of adolescence. Healthy children. 2019.
20. Palacios X. Adolescence: a problematic stage of human development? Revista Ciencias de la Salud. 2019;17:5-8.
21. Bernal Daisy H, Hevia Leisy P. Pregnancy and adolescence. Cuban Journal of Paediatrics. 2020;92.
22. Riquelme M, García OF, Serra E. Psychosocial maladjustment in adolescence: parental socialization, self-esteem and substance use. Anales de Psicología/Annals of Psychology. 2018;34(3):536-44.
23. Mazuera-Arias R, Albornoz-Arias N, Vivas-García M, Carreño-Paredes M-T, Cuberos M-A, Lalinde JDH, et al. Influence of sex education on adolescent motherhood in Táchira State, Venezuela. Archivos Venezolanos de Farmacología y Terapéutica. 2018;37(3):176-83.
24. Jacome-Gallegos CS, Parra-Torres SY, Paccha-Tamay CL. Factors influencing early pregnancy among adolescents in Pasaje, Ecuador. Polo del Conocimiento. 2021;6(7):1200-11.
25. Mariscal EMA, Puente AVG, Tobar LLO, Calderón JAM. Causes related to early pregnancy in adolescents in Babahoyo canton, province of Los Rios, Ecuador. Science and Education-Scientific Journal. 2020;1(8):6-16.
26. González DM, Loor ÁD, Briones SV, López L. Characterization of pregnancy in adolescents under 15 years of age attended in the primary health care area El Milagro, Riochico. QhaliKay Journal of Health Sciences ISSN: 2588-0608. 2021;5(2):8-16.
27. Ferrer Santos GE. Risk factors associated with sexually transmitted infections in pregnant adolescents attended at the rezola-cañete support hospital 2017. 2018.
28. Cos Hernández Y, Salazar B, Maylin2 Salgado Rodríguez K. Educational intervention on teenage pregnancy in the Reynaldo Castro complex. El Salvador Educational intervention on teenage pregnancy in the Reynaldo Castro complex. The Savior.
29. Zetina-Hernández E, Gerónimo-Carrillo R, Herrera-Castillo Y, de los Santos-Córdova L, Mirón-Hernández G. Preconception reproductive risk factors in women of childbearing age in a community in Tabasco. Salud Quintana Roo. 2018;11(40):7-10.

7 ANNEXES

ANNEX 1. INFORMED CONSENT FOR THE ADOLESCENT

Esperanza, of of 20__.

I, , hereby

I express my consent to participate as a research subject. I have been informed by the investigators of the purpose of the study and the manner in which it will be conducted. All the clarifications I have needed have been answered, and I have been assured that my identity will not be revealed. I can withdraw from the investigation at any time without any harm to myself. For the record, I sign this document in the presence of a witness:

Subject: . Signature: .

Witness: . Signature: .

Researcher: . Signature: .

ANNEX 2. INFORMED CONSENT FOR THE PARENT OR GUARDIAN OF THE CHILD

ADOLESCENT

Esperanza, of 20__.I, , do hereby

i express my consent for my daughter ,

participate as a subject in the research. I have been informed by the researchers of the purpose of the study and how it will be conducted. All the clarifications I have needed have been answered, and I have been given the assurance that your identity will not be revealed. You are free to withdraw from the investigation at any time, without any harm to yourself. For the record, I sign this document in the presence of a witness:

Subject: . Signature: .

Witness: . Signature: .

Researcher: . Signature: .

ANNEX 3. SURVEY

The information obtained in this questionnaire is for the exclusive use of the research staff, the data will be handled in aggregate and never individually. The choice in each question will be made by marking the corresponding line with an (x). Based on the results of this study, comprehensive health care programmes will be improved in terms of family planning with the aim of improving the sexual and reproductive health of adolescent girls.

We thank them for their cooperation in this research.

1: Age: ___ Age: ___ Age: ___ Age: ___ Age: ___ Age: ___

2: Schooling:

Primary___ Secondary Pre-university

3: Can you tell us at what age you had your first sexual intercourse?

4: - Currently you and your partner maintain: We are married, We are boyfriend and girlfriend, concubinage, I don't want to disclose__.

6- Have you experienced abortion or menstrual regulation?

a) Yes, No, I don't want to reveal it.

b) If yes, what was the main reason?

age, ___

other young children

peer pressure

family pressure

disruption of personal development

economic difficulties__.

housing difficulties

7: Do you know if there is a history of termination of pregnancy in your family?

Grandmother(s):

-Yes

-No

Mother:

-Yes

-No

Aunt(s):

-Yes

-No

Sister(s):

-Yes

-No

8: Within these Sexually Transmitted Infections, mark with an x if you have had or have had any of the following: HIV/AIDS. __. Blenorrhagia__. Syphilis__. Trichomonas__. Chlamydia__. Hepatitis B and C__. Herpes simplex__. Condyloma__. Unknown__.

9: Do you use contraception to protect yourself during sexual intercourse: Yes ___ No ___ Which ones?

Condom.

- D.I.U (copper tee, multiload, handle, ring)
- Tablets.
- Rhythm method.
- Coitus interruptus.

-Surgical sterilisation.

10- Do you usually drink alcohol? Never, Sometimes, Almost Always, Always, I don't want to reveal it.

Annex #4 FF-SIL Test

Almost	Little	A	Much	Almost

nunc a	s times	times	s times	always e

1. Decisions are made for important family matters.

2. Harmony prevails in my house.
3. In my house everyone fulfils their responsibilities.
4. Expressions of affection are part of our daily lives.
5. We express ourselves without innuendo, clearly and directly.
6. We can accept the shortcomings of others and cope with them.
7. We take into consideration the experiences of other families in difficult situations.
8. When someone in the family has a problem, the others help them.
9. Tasks are distributed in such a way that no one is overburdened.
10. Family customs can be modified
certain situations.
11. We can discuss various topics without fear.
12. Faced with a difficult family situation, we are able to seek help from others.
13. The interests and needs of each individual are respected by the family unit.
14. We show each other how fond we are of each other.

Scale values

Almost always5
Many4
times
Sometimes3
Rarely2
Almost never1

Diagnosis of family functioning according to FF-SIL total score

Functional	From 70 to 57 points
Moderately functional	From56 to 43 points
Dysfunctional	From42 to 28 points
Severely dysfunctional	From27 to 14 points

ANNEX 5. KNOWLEDGE QUESTIONNAIRE:

1: Do you think pregnancy at your age is risky?

a) Yes, my organism is not fully developed.
b) Yes, although my organism is already fit, but I have no conditions.
c) No, I have all the conditions and my parents help me with the upbringing.
to continue my studies.
d) Yes, I am not ready to have a child in any sense of my life.
e) No, I have a steady partner who is older than me and supports me.
economically.

f) No, it's a way of getting out of my parents, now they can't say anything, I have become an adult.

g) No, my friends have gotten pregnant and have not had any problems, besides.

that helps to support the couple.

h) Yes, although my friends were not harmed, their health was put at risk, as well as the health and safety of their friends.

of the baby.

i) It doesn't do any harm to give birth early, it's even better because I get out of it quickly.

j) If I get pregnant, my studies will be interrupted.

k) I don't know.

2- -Some young people mix alcohol consumption with sex. What do you think this can lead to?

a) I lose control over myself.

b) Sometimes I forget to use a condom.

c) I like it because I disinhibit myself and enjoy the relationship better.

d) I am more exposed to infection.

e) It's very nice to have sex with a few too many drinks.

f) I don't know.

3- What causes do you think can lead to a teenage girl becoming pregnant?

a) Not having a condom.

b) Linking alcohol and sex.

c) Wanting to get pregnant in order to leave home.

d) Wanting to study.

e) To be part of a family that understands her.

f) Not having a lot of money.

g) Be very knowledgeable about sexuality education.

h) Being the daughter of a teenage mother.

i) I don't know.

4- What harms can teenage pregnancy cause?

a) Many of my friends have become pregnant and it doesn't cause them any problems.

damage.

b) Sometimes they feel sad.

c) Many families do not help them.

d) They grow old quickly in the boy's care.

e) They can almost always support the couple, as a child helps to keep the couple together.

relationship becomes more real

f) There are no problems with the school.

g) Often the family does not want the pregnancy and they have to abort the pregnancy at the time of

child.

h) The risks that adolescents face with pregnancy are the following same for all women.

i) Children of adolescent girls are born in better conditions than those of adolescent boys.

other mothers.

j) Adolescent girls are more anaemic during pregnancy.

k) I don't know.

5- What health harms can an abortion cause? Name a few:

6- What do you think about condom use in sexual relations?

a) It protects me from pregnancy.

b) It diminishes the pleasure of the relationship.

c) Protects against sexual infections.

d) There's no way I'm going to propose to men, they always say that no.

e) I haven't even learned how to use it, that's a man's job.

f) I don't know.

Instructions

Question	Expected response	Qualification
1	Subparagraphs a, d, h and j.	Five points for each positive response. Total: 20 points.
2	Subparagraphs a, b and d.	5 points for each good answer or for each positive answer. Total: 15 points.
3	Sub-paragraphs a, b, c, f, h,	4 points for each positive answer. Total: 20 points
4	Subparagraphs b, c, d, g .	5 points for each positive answer. Total: 20 points
5	By his words he alludes to ovarian debris, endometritis, infections, haemorrhages, uterine perforation; psychological damage such as anxiety, depression, avoidance, rejection of the environment; and social damage such as disruption of the teaching process, school rejection, rejection	One point for each positive answer. Total: 5 points.

	by peers, lack of family support.	
6	Subparagraphs a and c.	Ten points for each positive response. Total: 20 points.
Overall rating 100 points	Good: 80 points and more.	
	Regular: 70-79 points.	
	Bad: Less than 70 points.	

ANNEX 6. EDUCATIONAL PROGRAMME

1-General:

The educational programme will be aimed at female adolescents belonging to CMF 5 of the Mario Muñoz Monroy polyclinic in the town of Esperanza, in the municipality of Ranchuelo, taking 35 patients belonging to the same as a sample for the study. It will be carried out in the period between February 2020-February 2022. The contents to be addressed will be according to the individual and group diagnosis in order to enrich the knowledge about adolescent pregnancy and to control the modifiable risk factors associated with it.

2-Substantiation:

Aimed at female adolescents in CMF 5 of the Mario Muñoz Monroy polyclinic in the town of Esperanza. Observation reveals deficiencies in the quality of health promotion and prevention activities for adolescent girls. There is insufficient knowledge of the modifiable risk factors associated with adolescent pregnancy, which favours the appearance of pregnancy in this population and the appearance of complications, also determined by inadequate control of these modifiable risk factors. In order to offer a solution to this problematic situation, the author proposes an educational programme for the prevention and control of modifiable risk factors in adolescents that influence the appearance of adolescent pregnancy.

3-Objective General:

Develop an adolescent education programme that enables the recognition of modifiable risk factors associated with adolescent pregnancy.

4-Content:

Dosage of topics:

No. of the subject.	Duration.
1: Introduction to the educational programme.	1hour
2: Adolescence. Definition and main characteristics.	1hour
3: Sexuality and reproductive risk.	1 hour
4: Adolescent pregnancy. Causes of adolescent pregnancy.	1 hour
5: Consequences of adolescent pregnancy.	1 hour
6: Consequences of abortion.	1 hour
7: Contraceptive methods.	1 hour
8: Condom use.	1 hour
9: Sexually transmitted infections.	1 hour
10: Consequences of alcohol consumption associated with relationships !s.	1 hour
11 : Final evaluation of the educational programme.	1 hour

Methodological guidelines

In order to achieve significant learning of the aforementioned contents and objectives, we will develop an educational process with several group sessions, using different active pedagogical techniques such as exposition, video with discussion, analysis of situations, among others.

6-Evaluation:

The evaluation of the educational programme will be carried out from two perspectives:

-To know whether the proposed objectives have been achieved.

-Determine whether the activities outlined in the programme have been carried out as expected.

Evaluation will take place throughout the intervention process: before, during and at the end:

Before implementing the educational programme

The first assessment will be carried out before starting the intervention by applying a questionnaire (see Annex 4), individual diagnosis of learning needs and group diagnosis through analysis and expository techniques for carrying out the general consolidation assessment and the elaboration of the educational diagnosis.

During the implementation of the educational programme

The evaluation of the process will be participatory as an active subject, through the procedures of self-evaluation, co-evaluation and heteroevaluation in each activity.

After the educational programme has been implemented

At the end of the programme, a second evaluation will be carried out to assess changes in the level of information and the same instrument used before starting the intervention will be applied.

The evaluation of the indicators and variables identified to measure the effectiveness of the intervention will be carried out, specifying the period to be evaluated and comparing the results BEFORE and AFTER, according to the health problem that was the object of the research and the modifiable factors.

Session 1. Introduction to the Education Programme

Objectives: To introduce the members of the group.

To determine the level of knowledge about adolescent pregnancy.

To know the expectations of the group in relation to the topics to be addressed.

Relax the group.

Introduction: "El patio de mi casa" technique.

Objective: to enable the subjects to get to know each other.

Procedure: form two circles, one inside the other. Both circles are guided to go around and the people facing each other will introduce themselves. They are guided to take a step and so on until everyone has been introduced.

Development: The Expectations Technique.

Objective: to identify the group's expectations about the issues to be addressed.

Procedure: each member is given a sheet of paper and asked the following questions:

- What do I expect to find from these activities?
- What issues will be addressed and how will I feel about them?
- What will I take away from these activities?

Once this has been done individually and anonymously, the sheets are mixed in a box and each participant takes one at random and reads it aloud to the whole group. The sheets remain on a table set up for this purpose and can be evaluated at the end of the application.

Apply the knowledge questionnaire.

Conclusions: Hand out cards with a problem situation to be discussed at the next meeting.

Time: 60 minutes.

Session 2. Adolescence. Definition and characteristics.

Objectives:

-Reflect on the particularities of adolescence and its definition.

-Defining adolescence.

-Describe the physical and psychological characteristics of adolescents.

Introduction: "Food for Life" technique.

Objective: to raise the self-esteem of the group members.

Procedure: third person sentences are given to each participant to read in the first person.

Example: "You are a very talented person". The participant should read "I am a person...".

The following are suggested phrases that can be used.

- You speak well.

- You are smart.
- You know how to make others feel good.
- You are creative.
- You have a personal magnetism.
- People admire your patience and tolerance.
- You know how to lead a life.
- You have a beautiful soul.
- People are looking for you.
- You are a person who loves others.

Development: Technique "Talking about my adolescence".

Objectives:

-Create a sense of cohesion and group spirit.

-To highlight anxieties and fears that prevent discussion of sexuality in adolescence. Encourage mutual trust. Explain and define adolescence.

Procedure: form subgroups of four people, who will have to talk to each other about a humorous experience with sexual content that occurred in adolescence (it can be personal or someone else's, without identifying it); at the end, each group chooses the one they consider most important or most humorous, to tell it to the rest of the participants.

If the group is large, ask two subgroups (eight people) to come back together to form a larger group and repeat the exercise they did in the original subgroup.

Talking points:

- Was it difficult to think about the experience they had to tell?
- How did they feel to their peers about the experience?
- Of the experiences mentioned, were most of them: personal, third party, jokes?

Evaluation: co-evaluation.

Conclusions: Establish a knowledge encounter "who knows more, reads more", aimed at adolescents learning more about adolescence and recognising the main risk factors and their impact on quality of life.

Session 3. Sexuality and reproductive risk.

Objective:

-To promote the appropriation of information on sexuality in adolescence and preconceptional reproductive risk. Discuss preconceptional reproductive risk at this stage.

Introduction: "What do I see?

In front of a mirror, the participants observe their faces and describe them, focusing on the different structures, and compare themselves with each other. After this, they are given some accessories and are encouraged to put them on, then they are asked: what or who do they look like with these elements on?

Development: "Psychodrama" technique.

This technique allows the diagnosis of a group's educational needs in a given situation, motivates the group to learn a technique or acquire new knowledge. The application is based on the observation of a real fact or situation; in this particular case, sexuality in adolescence is addressed from the female perspective and reproductive risk.

Conclusions: Technique "The handkerchief game".

Part of the assessment of the facial expressions of adolescents.

They are then asked what they do when they are sad and what they do when they are happy. When the handkerchief is thrown upwards, the participants imitate gestures of joy, and when it touches the ground, of sadness. Little by little, the whole body is incorporated into the expressions.

Finally, the group members are asked to draw together some happy faces and one sad face.

Evaluation: Co-evaluation.

Session 4. Adolescent pregnancy. Definition and causes.

Objectives:

-Defining adolescent pregnancy.

-Determine the causes of adolescent pregnancy.

Introduction: Technique "Sounds that surround me".

The facilitator asks the adolescents to close their eyes and listen to sounds coming from outside, e.g. in the other room, in the street, in the courtyard, etc. The facilitator then asks the adolescents individually to mention some of the sounds they heard, and to try to imitate or reproduce them. The adolescents are then asked individually to mention some of the sounds they heard, and to try to imitate or reproduce them. Emphasis should be placed on sounds coming from nature in order to establish a link with the subsequent technique.

Development: "Problem tree" technique.

Objective: to identify causes and effects of a problem.

Procedure: The group is instructed to draw a tree on a flipchart or poster board, or on a blackboard. The facilitator will place the problem (teenage pregnancy) on the trunk of the tree, and the participants will write down the causes of the problem on the roots and the consequences on the leaves, emphasising health.

In general, possible solutions to this problem will be discussed.

Evaluation: Co-evaluation.

Conclusions: Clarify all the questions on the topic taught.

Session 5. Consequences of adolescent pregnancy.

Objective:

-Discuss the consequences of teenage pregnancy.

Introduction: "Masks" technique.

The facilitator talks about some masks she made for this working session, which she

has stored in a bag (this should be occupied as if it were really full).
Sitting in a circle, he shows the teenagers the masks, which he carefully takes out of the bag. They will soon discover that they are just imagination. However, the facilitator shows them how to put them on their face, while doing this step they can add accessories on their face or make funny gestures.
Then encourage the adolescents to each choose a mask from the bag and put it on.
Development: "La Balanza" technique.
Objectives: to stimulate participants to learn how to think and decide whether or not to bear children during adolescence.
Materials: sheet of paper and pencil.
Procedure: A sheet of paper is given to the subjects undergoing training and they are asked to write down all the advantages and disadvantages for them:

- Being pregnant.
- Not be pregnant.

The individual debate proceeds where the individual motive and direction of the balance is decided, as well as the attitude to be decided.
Conclusions: Technique "Let's get into the picture".
The facilitator stimulates the participants, previously dividing the group in two, to represent a "tableau". One of them will represent pregnant adolescents. In the other, non-pregnant adolescents will be represented.
After all participants are inside the 'box', they have to say how they feel inside it. The activity ends by comparing one "box" with the other.
Evaluation: Co-evaluation
Session 6. Abortion.
Explain abortion as a contraceptive method, its causes and consequences.
Introduction: "What am I doing right? What am I doing wrong?" technique.
Objective: to stimulate the subjects to reflect on different attitudes towards life, which do or do not favour personal and collective well-being.
Materials: blackboard, chalk and banner.
Procedure: Introduce the activity by talking about positive and negative behaviours in relation to sexual practices in adolescence. Each person will have their own criteria and together they will come to know what the general criteria of the group is. The participants are informed that they have 5 minutes to think about good and bad behaviours in relation to sexual practices at this stage of life. Afterwards, they will brainstorm their views, which the coordinator will write on the blackboard; first, what is good on the left and then, what is bad, on the right. Subjects will be asked to reflect on the similar criteria in order to group them together and arrive at the group's general criterion, which will be formed into a banner.
Development: Dramatisation technique for consequences of abortion.
Objective: Reflection on consequences and behavioural changes in relation to

abortion.

Procedure: nine volunteers are selected from the group and given the following roles: a 15-year-old female adolescent, a 16-year-old male adolescent (played by a girl from the group), the parents of both adolescents, a teacher and 2 friends (a friend for the female and a friend for the supposed male).

The adolescent is informed of the possibility of pregnancy and the intention to have an abortion, which she has to communicate to her boyfriend.

It must be represented:

- Reaction from both.
- Then, the reaction of the teenager and her friend.
- Then, the reaction of the teenager and his friend.
- The teenager then asks her teacher for advice.
- Then, the teenager with her mother, then, confronting both parents.
- Confrontation of the adolescent with his mother, who found out about it through comments, and later, the adolescent with his parents.
- Participants' position on the suggestion of abortion. Its causes and consequences.

Talking points:

- What happens at each step of the dramatisation?
- What do group members think of each situation?

At the end of the technique, adolescents' self-esteem and confidence will be strengthened to facilitate a proper understanding of the consequences of their decisions.

Conclusions: The "Three Chairs" technique

Objective: to assess the results of group work for educational purposes.

Procedure: three chairs are placed in the centre of a circle where all the members of the group are situated. Each chair is marked with a sign:

- How did I get here?
- How did I feel?
- How do I leave?

Each person in turn will occupy the three chairs and express their feelings according to the instructions. To close the exercise, a collective creation reflecting the general feelings can be made in the form of a Collective Poem. Each person writes a poetic phrase about the exercises and gives it to some people designated by their literary attitudes to make the group composition. No phrases should be changed, just arranged artistically and given a title using one of them.

It will be read animatedly to the whole group.

Session 7. Preventing adolescent pregnancy. Use of contraceptive methods.

Objectives:

-To analyse the situations and conflicts experienced by adolescent girls at the

beginning of their sexual life.
-Reflect on the risks of irresponsible sexual behaviour.
Development:
-Opening: Commentary on the previous meeting.
-Presentation of the theme: Active sexual life. Contraceptive methods.
Exchange views on the importance of protected sexual activity to avoid pregnancy and also STIs.
-Discuss the importance of condom use.
Closing: Completing incomplete sentences.
Conclusions: Clarify all the questions on the topic taught.
Technique: Group discussion.
Evaluation: Co-evaluation
Duration: 60 minutes.
Session 8. Condom use in the prevention of adolescent pregnancy and STIs.
Objective: To encourage condom use in sexual relations.
Introduction: "Telegram" technique.
Objective: group animation.
Procedure: the audience sits in a circle and a member of the group comes out with the telegram, which gives the key to change seats, it can be for external aspects, colour of clothes, shoes, etcetera. Whoever loses (is left without a seat), repeats the same thing.
Example: I received a telegram saying: "everyone with black shoes should change their chairs". Start with general aspects and then include those related to sexuality in adolescence. For example: "everyone who does not always use a condom during sex should change chairs...".
Development: "Fears and Hopes" technique.
Objective: to eliminate doubts and fears that arise as a result of the use of condoms in sexual relations.
Procedure: the participants express their fears and fears in some particularities of their own. These are discussed in the group, which tries to find a solution.
Technique "The stars".
To develop this technique you need cardboard stars with questions on the theme. The stars are glued on cardboard or paper to resemble a firmament. Each participant is asked to take a star and answer the question on it.
The questions will ask about adolescent sexuality and condom use.
Session 9. Sexually Transmitted Infections
Objectives:
-Explain about the main sexually transmitted infections.
-Influencing a responsible attitude towards sexuality.
Development:

Presentation of the theme.

We will cover the most common sexually transmitted infections such as syphilis, blennorrhoea, HIV-AIDS, genital herpes, among others, as well as their clinical picture and ways to prevent them.

Technique: Group discussion.

Evaluation: Co-evaluation.

Conclusions: Explain any remaining unexplained doubts raised in the discussion and hand out questions related to the next meeting.

Session 10. Alcohol consumption and sexual relations.

Objective: To determine the consequences of alcohol intake associated with sexual intercourse.

Development: "What am I doing right? What am I doing wrong?" technique.

Objective: to stimulate the subjects to reflect on different attitudes towards life, which may or may not favour personal or collective well-being.

Materials: blackboard, chalk and banner.

Procedure: Introduce the activity by talking about positive and negative behaviours in relation to sexual practices in adolescence, especially the association between alcohol and sexual intercourse. Each person will have their own criteria and together they will come to know what the general criteria of the group is. The subjects are informed that they have 5 minutes to think about good and bad behaviours in relation to sexual practices at this stage of life. Afterwards, they will brainstorm their views, which the coordinator will write on the blackboard; first, what is good on the left and then, what is bad on the right. Subjects will be asked to reflect on the similar criteria in order to group them together and arrive at the group's general criteria, which will be formed into a banner.

Evaluation: Co-evaluation.

Conclusions: Cards will be handed out with writings about alcohol consumption and its impact on sexual and reproductive health.

Session 11. Final evaluation of the educational programme.

Objective: To determine the level of knowledge about adolescent pregnancy.

Technique "Leave your heavy load here and pick up your joy".

Objectives: to reduce fears and hopelessness in relation to teenage pregnancy, and to enable the expression of positive feelings.

Materials: pencil, paper, boxes with positive sentences on how to control the problematic situation.

Procedure: Participants are asked to write on a piece of paper something that causes them concern in relation to sexuality and teenage pregnancy, which is poured into a box that is closed and thrown away. Then another box is taken with small pieces of paper expressing positive situations and feelings related to the development of responsible and happy sexuality at this stage.

This will be followed by the knowledge questionnaire applied at the beginning of the educational programme.
Conclusions: Closing the intervention.

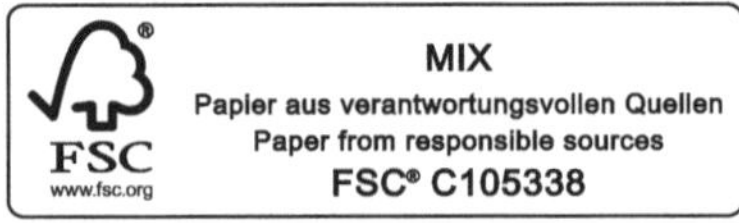

Printed by Books on Demand GmbH, Norderstedt / Germany